BREASTFEEDING BONDS
SUPERHEROES: EMPOWERING THE JOURNEY
Unleashing the Superpowers of Motherhood for a Thriving Future

DR. DALAL AKOURY

Copyright © 2023 Dr. Dalal Akoury

BREASTFEEDING BONDS

All rights reserved. No part of this publication may be reproduced, distributed, or transmitted in any form or by any means, including photocopying, recording, or other electronic or mechanical methods, without the prior written permission of the publisher, except in the case of brief quotations embodied in critical reviews and certain other noncommercial uses permitted by copyright law. For permission requests, write to the publisher, addressed "Attention: Permissions Coordinator," at info@beyondpublishing.net

Quantity sales and special discounts are available on quantity purchases by corporations, associations, and others. For details, contact the publisher at the address above.

Orders by U.S. trade bookstores and wholesalers. Email info@BeyondPublishing.net

The Beyond Publishing Speakers Bureau can bring authors to your live event. For more information or to book an event contact the Beyond Publishing Speakers Bureau speak@BeyondPublishing.net

The Author can be reached directly at BeyondPublishing.net

Manufactured and printed in the United States of America distributed globally by BeyondPublishing.net

New York | Los Angeles | London | Sydney

ISBN Softcover: 978-1-63792-637-6
ISBN Hardcover: 978-1-63792-628-4

TABLE OF CONTENTS

Foreword   8

Chapter 1: The Wonders of Breast Milk   10
- The composition of breast milk
- Nutritional benefits for infants
- Unique antibodies and immune-boosting properties

Chapter 2: Breastfeeding: A Journey Begins   14
- The importance of breastfeeding initiation
- The first latch and establishing breastfeeding
- Overcoming initial challenges

Chapter 3: Breastfeeding and Maternal Health   20
- Physical and emotional benefits for breastfeeding mothers
- The role of breastfeeding in postpartum recovery
- Long-term health benefits for mothers

Chapter 4: Bonding through Breastfeeding   24
- The emotional connection between mother and child
- Oxytocin release and its impact on bonding
- Promoting secure attachment through breastfeeding

Chapter 5: Breastfeeding and Childhood Health   28
- The long-term health benefits of breastfeeding
- Reduced risk of infections, allergies, and chronic diseases
- Cognitive development and IQ benefits

Chapter 6: Breastfeeding Challenges and Solutions   31
- Common breastfeeding challenges and how to address them
- Seeking support from lactation consultants and support groups

- Tips for managing breastfeeding difficulties

Chapter 7: Expressing and Storing Breast Milk   35
- Benefits of expressing breast milk
- Different methods of expressing milk (manual, electric pumps)
- Proper storage and handling of expressed breast milk

Chapter 8: Breastfeeding and the Working Mother   38
- Balancing breastfeeding with returning to work
- Strategies for pumping at work and maintaining milk supply
- Legal protections and workplace accommodations

Chapter 9: Breastfeeding and Society   42
- Promoting a breastfeeding-friendly society
- Addressing social stigma and public perception
- Breastfeeding support resources and initiatives

Chapter 10: Celebrating the Breastfeeding Journey   46
- Reflecting on the personal stories of breastfeeding mothers
- Recognizing the joys and challenges of breastfeeding
- Words of encouragement and inspiration for breastfeeding mothers

Chapter 11: Breastfeeding and the Support Network   50
- The power of peer support
- Uniting forces for success
- Pillars of support

Chapter 12: Breastfeeding and Society   54
- Shattering stereotypes and changing narratives
- Activism for breastfeeding rights

- Celebrating a breastfeeding-friendly society

Chapter 13: Inspiring Generations 58
- Passing the torch
- The ripple effect
- The superhero legacy

Acknowledgements 62
Ressources and Support 66
References 68
About the Author 70
Final Thoughts 72

FOREWORD

DR. DEB MATTHEW

Have you ever witnessed the incredible power of breastfeeding? Have you marveled at the unbreakable bond between a mother and her child as they embark on this remarkable journey together? Prepare to be captivated by "Breastfeeding Superheroes: Empowering the Journey."

In this book, Dr. Dalal Akoury takes you on a transformative exploration of the super heroic world of breastfeeding. As a renowned expert in the field, Dr. Akoury brings a wealth of knowledge, compassion, and experience to every page. She sheds light on the physical, emotional, and psychological benefits of breastfeeding, highlighting its profound impact on the lives of both mother and baby.

Through heartfelt stories, evidence-based information, and practical guidance, Dr. Akoury celebrates the strength, resilience, and love that breastfeeding superheroes embody. She invites you to witness the magic of breast milk, the power of the mother-child connection, and the transformative journey of empowerment that awaits.

As you delve into these pages, you will gain a deeper understanding of the unique qualities of breast milk and its ability to nourish, protect, and nurture. Dr. Akoury guides you through the triumphs and challenges of breastfeeding, offering invaluable insights and empowering strategies to support your own breastfeeding superhero journey.

Prepare to be inspired, encouraged, and uplifted. This book is a celebration of the extraordinary bond between mother and baby, a testament to the strength of every breastfeeding superhero, and a source of guidance and inspiration for mothers worldwide. I am honored to introduce you to this empowering book, written by a true advocate for breastfeeding superheroes. Dr. Dalal Akoury's passion, expertise, and commitment shine through every word, providing a beacon of light for mothers on their breastfeeding journey.

Embrace your inner superhero. Embrace the power of breastfeeding. Let the journey begin.

CHAPTER 1

THE MAGICAL ELIXIR: UNVEILING THE WONDERS OF BREAST MILK

Quote:

"Breastfeeding is an extraordinary journey, where love and nourishment intertwine to create a powerful force of nature. A mother's embrace becomes a source of unwavering strength, forging an unbreakable bond. Embrace the profound impact of breastfeeding and let it shape a future filled with love, resilience, and boundless possibilities."

Once upon a time, in a world of tiny miracles, there exists a magical elixir called breast milk. Its journey begins deep within a mother's body, where it transforms into a mesmerizing concoction that nurtures and empowers infants in the most enchanting ways. Join us as we embark on an immersive journey into the realm of breast milk, where vibrant colors and vivid landscapes bring its wonders to life.

1.1 The Symphony of Nutrients: A Harmonious Blend

Picture an orchestra of colors and textures swirling together in perfect harmony. Breast milk is a symphony of nutrients, orchestrated to meet the precise needs of a growing baby. Imagine vibrant hues of golden colostrum, rich in antibodies and immune-boosting properties, gradually transitioning to creamy milk filled with essential carbohydrates, proteins, fats, vitamins, minerals, and enzymes. These nutrients dance together,

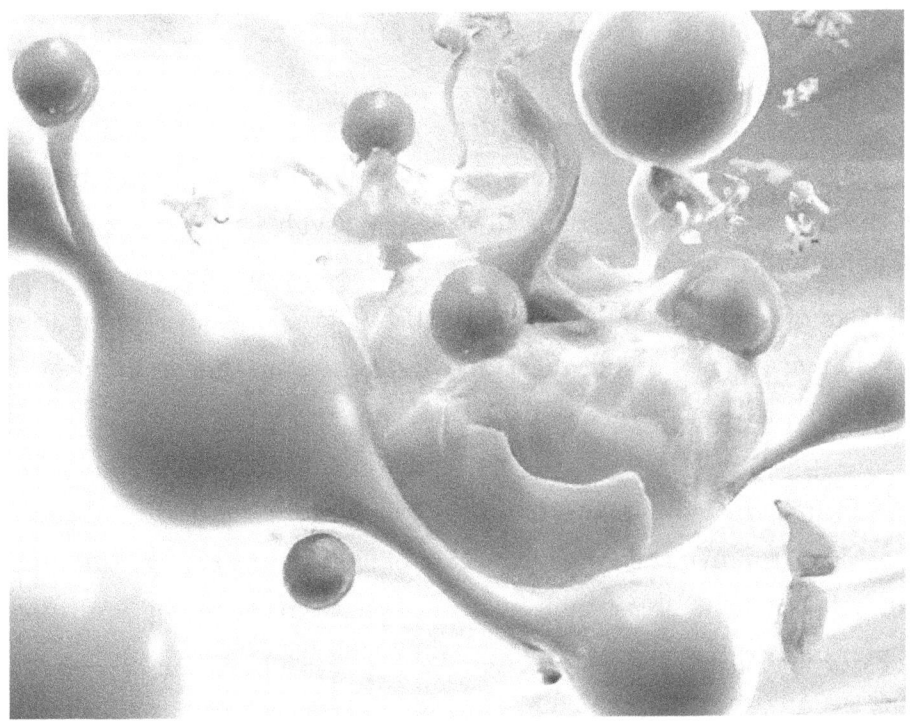

like the harmonious notes of a symphony, nurturing the baby's body and fostering optimal development.

1.2 The Superpowers Within: Defenders of Health

Step into a magical realm where tiny superheroes come to life. Breast milk is no ordinary liquid—it possesses extraordinary superpowers! Visualize a legion of antibodies, immune cells, and protective substances forming an impenetrable shield around the baby, defending against harmful invaders. These superheroes are the guardians of health, ensuring the baby's well-being and safeguarding against the forces of illness and infection.

1.3 A Journey of Digestive Delight: From Flavorful Exploration to Nourishing Absorption

Imagine a whimsical garden of flavors, bursting with fruits, vegetables, and delightful surprises. Breast milk takes babies on an extraordinary journey of digestive delight. With its unique blend of enzymes, prebiotics, and friendly probiotics, breast milk serves as a garden of nourishment. Visualize the baby's taste buds awakening to a symphony of flavors, while their tiny digestive system effortlessly absorbs the nutrients, leaving them satisfied and content.

1.4 From Tiny Fighters to Victorious Champions: Building Resilience

Enter a mythical kingdom where brave warriors emerge from the tiniest of beings. Breast milk becomes their secret weapon, bestowing upon them extraordinary strength and resilience. Like a suit of armor, breast milk fortifies premature and sick babies, nurturing their fragile organs, bolstering their immune systems, and shielding them from common challenges. These babies transform into champions, conquering the hurdles before them and emerging victorious.

1.5 Love, Bonding, and Magic: An Unbreakable Connection

In the realm of breastfeeding, love, and bonding weave a tapestry of enchantment. Picture a serene garden, where mother and baby sit amidst a symphony of fragrant flowers. As the baby nestles close, the act of breastfeeding releases a magical hormone called oxytocin. This love potion fills the air, enveloping mother, and child in an ethereal embrace. Their hearts beat in synchrony, and an unbreakable bond form, filled with warmth, tenderness, and an unspoken connection that is as powerful as any spell.

Conclusion:

In this captivating chapter, we have unveiled the secrets of breast milk—the magical elixir that nurtures and empowers our little heroes. Its symphony of nutrients, the superpowers of immunity, the journey of digestive delight, and the ability to foster love and bonding make it a truly enchanting potion. Breast milk paints a vibrant canvas of nourishment, resilience, and unbreakable connections in the wondrous journey of infancy.

In our next chapter, we will follow the footsteps of mothers and babies as they embark on their extraordinary breastfeeding adventure. Prepare to be captivated by the dance of nurturing and the bonds that blossom, as we explore the art of breastfeeding and the magical moments it brings.

CHAPTER 2

THE DANCE OF NURTURING: EMBRACING THE ART OF BREASTFEEDING

Quote:

"Celebrate the breastfeeding journey as a symphony of love and resilience, where a mother's body orchestrates the most extraordinary nourishment for her child. Each latch, each precious moment, weaves a tapestry of connection, fostering a bond that transcends time. Embrace the power of breastfeeding and witness the harmony it creates, nurturing both body and soul."

As the sun rises in the sky, a gentle breeze whispers through the leaves, signaling the beginning of a new chapter—a chapter filled with the artistry and magic of breastfeeding. In this enchanting realm, mothers and babies embark on a dance of nurturing, where love, connection, and nourishment intertwine. Join us as we unveil the captivating steps of this extraordinary journey, brought to life through animated tales and vibrant visuals.

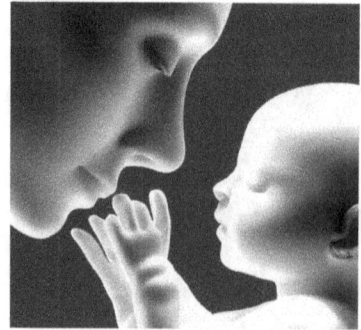

2.1 The Dance Begins: Initiating the Bond

Imagine a stage bathed in soft, warm hues as a mother and her baby take center stage. With tender grace, the mother cradles her baby in her arms, ready to embark on the dance of nurturing. The first latch is like the opening note of a beautiful melody, setting the stage for a harmonious connection between mother and child.

2.2 The Rhythm of Synchronization: Finding the Perfect Tempo

The dance continues as mother and baby find their rhythm—a synchronization of movements that brings them closer together. The baby's tiny hands explore, gently grasping the mother's finger, while their eyes meet in an exchange of love and trust. The mother's body responds, producing milk in perfect harmony with the baby's needs, ensuring an abundant supply of nourishment.

2.3 The Power of Skin-to-Skin: A Tender Embrace

Enter a realm of warmth and closeness, where skin-to-skin contact creates a magical bond between mother and baby. As they embrace, the mother's body responds, releasing a surge of oxytocin—the love hormone—flooding both of them with feelings of comfort and tranquility. This intimate connection strengthens the dance, deepening the bond and creating a safe space for the baby to thrive.

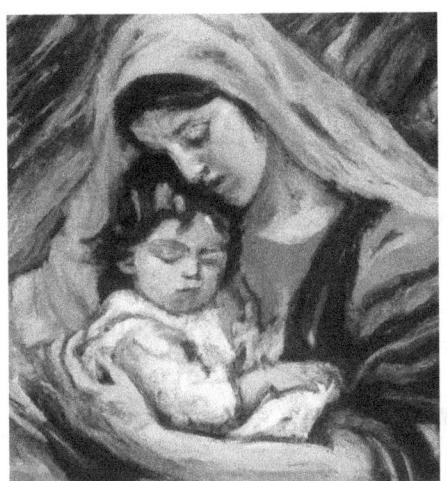

2.4 The Art of Positioning: A Symphony of Comfort

In this animated realm, the mother becomes a master of positioning, guiding her baby into a symphony of comfortable postures. Visualize the baby nestled in the crook of the mother's arm, their bodies in perfect alignment. The mother's gentle touch and nurturing gaze create an atmosphere of safety, allowing the baby to feed peacefully and joyfully.

2.5 A Feast for the Senses: Exploring the Flavors

The dance of nurturing becomes a feast for the senses, as the baby explores the flavors of breast milk. Each drop is a burst of sweetness, like a delectable treat from nature's pantry. The baby's delicate taste buds awaken to a symphony of tastes, while their satisfied expressions paint a vivid picture of contentment and delight.

2.6 The Dance of Comfort: Soothing and Nurturing

In this animated realm, breastfeeding becomes a soothing dance, comforting both mother and baby. Visualize the mother's loving gaze, her voice soft and soothing like a lullaby. As the baby suckles, their rhythmic movements become a gentle sway, creating a serene and peaceful atmosphere. This dance of comfort embraces their souls, creating moments of deep connection and tranquility.

Conclusion:

In this captivating chapter, we have witnessed the artistry and magic of breastfeeding—the dance of nurturing between mother and baby. Through animated tales and vibrant visuals, we have explored the initiation of the bond, the synchronization of movements, the power of skin-to-skin contact, the art of positioning, the exploration of flavors, and the dance of comfort. This mesmerizing journey showcases the depth of connection and love that blossom through the art of breastfeeding.

In the next chapter, we will embark on an adventure through the magical benefits of breastfeeding, uncovering the extraordinary ways it supports the baby's health and well-being. Prepare to be amazed by the wonders that breast milk holds within its embrace.

Breastfeeding Unveiled: The Dance of Nurturing

Welcome to the mesmerizing world of breastfeeding, where a magical dance unfolds between mother and baby. In this chapter, we invite you to witness the enchantment as they embark on a remarkable journey of connection, nourishment, and pure joy. Through vibrant animations and captivating storytelling, we delve into the art of breastfeeding, transforming it into a delightful and immersive experience.

2.7 The Symphony of Latch: A Graceful Ballet

Imagine stepping into a grand theater, the curtains drawing open to reveal a beautiful ballet performance. The act of latching during breastfeeding is no different—it is a dance of grace and synchrony. Watch as the baby instinctively seeks their mother's breast, guided by nature's wisdom. With gentle precision, they find their way, their tiny hands and mouths creating a tender connection that sets the stage for a nourishing embrace.

2.8 The Dance of Suckle: Rhythm and Harmony

Picture a joyous dance floor filled with laughter, rhythm, and boundless energy. As the baby latches onto the breast, they engage in a rhythmic motion of suckling. Their mouths move in perfect harmony, creating a delightful symphony of nourishment. The dance of suckle is not merely a physical act—it is a source of comfort, contentment, and the purest expression of trust and connection between mother and baby.

2.9 Nutritional Pas de Deux: A Feast for the Senses Imagine a lavish banquet table, adorned with an array of delicious delicacies.

Breast milk flows effortlessly, like a sparkling fountain of nourishment. Within its magical embrace, essential nutrients, antibodies, and enzymes perform a pas de deux, providing the baby with optimal nutrition and immune support. Witness the baby's satisfaction as they nourish their growing body, and marvel at the seamless partnership between mother and breast milk—an exquisite symphony of sustenance.

2.11 The Choreography of Bonding: A Garden of Love Envision a serene garden, where flowers bloom and emotions intertwine.

Breastfeeding is not only about nourishment but also a profound expression of love and bonding. As the baby feeds, an invisible thread weaves between their hearts, creating an unbreakable connection. Embrace the tender gaze between mother and baby—a language of love that transcends words. In this garden of love, their souls dance together, bound by an everlasting bond nurtured through breastfeeding.

2.12 The Symphony of Hormones: Harmonizing Emotions Step into a magical realm where hormones dance and sway, orchestrating emotions and bonding.

As the baby suckles, the mother's body releases a symphony of hormones. Oxytocin, the love hormone, surges through their veins, creating a sense of peace, calm, and an overwhelming feeling of love. Serotonin, the happiness hormone, fills the air with joy and contentment. This harmonious dance of hormones deepens the bond between mother and baby, enhancing the magical experience of breastfeeding.

2.13 The Joyful Cadence of Milk: Nurturing Rhythm Imagine a rhythmic melody playing in the background—a joyful cadence that accompanies each feeding session.

Breast milk flows in perfect synchrony, responding to the baby's needs in real-time. It ebbs and flows, adapting its composition to meet the growing demands of the baby. This rhythmic exchange of love and nourishment creates a sense of security and trust, enhancing the magical dance between mother and baby.

Conclusion:

In this captivating chapter, we have unveiled the artistry of breastfeeding—the dance of nurturing that unfolds between mother and baby. From the symphony of latch to the dance of suckle, each movement is a testament to the magical connection and nourishment shared. Witness the nutritional pas de deux, the choreography of bonding, and the symphony of hormones that elevate breastfeeding to a realm of wonder. Breastfeeding becomes a wondrous dance, where love, nourishment, and unbreakable bonds intertwine.

In our next chapter, we will explore the benefits of breastfeeding, uncovering the remarkable impact it has on the baby's health, development, and overall well-being. Get ready to witness the transformative power of breast milk in promoting a thriving and radiant start in life—a journey filled with boundless possibilities.

CHAPTER 3

BREASTFEEDING SUPERPOWERS: UNLEASHING A WORLD OF BENEFITS

Quote:
"Breastfeeding is a dance of love, where every rhythm and movement tell a unique story. It's a celebration of connection, as mother and child move in perfect harmony, nourishing both body and soul. Let the music of breastfeeding guide you on a journey of profound bonding, resilience, and the purest expression of maternal love.

Welcome to a world where breastfeeding unleashes a realm of superpowers for both mother and baby. In this action-packed chapter, we invite you to discover the extraordinary benefits that breastfeeding bestows upon them. Prepare to be dazzled by vibrant animations, interactive storytelling, and jaw-dropping feats of super heroic proportions as we explore the realm of breastfeeding superpowers.

3.1 Immunity Shield: The Power of Antibodies

Picture a fortress, guarded by an elite team of microscopic superheroes. Breast milk equips babies with an unrivaled immunity shield, powered by an army of antibodies. These tiny warriors, armed with capes made of immunoglobulins, swoop in to protect the baby from evil invaders like colds, flu, and pesky infections. They have the power to neutralize villains and keep the baby's immune system strong, creating a world where sniffles and sneezes dare not tread.

3.2 Brain Boosters: Fueling Cognitive Superpowers

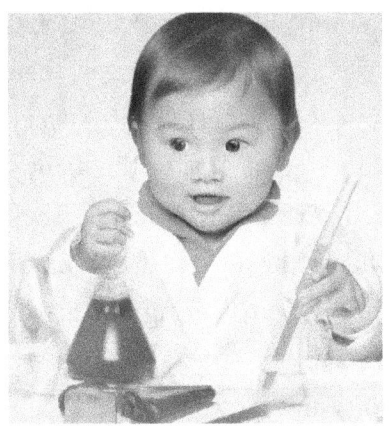

Imagine a laboratory filled with bubbling beakers and sparking electrical circuits. Breast milk contains a mind-boggling concoction of brain boosters that would make even the most brilliant scientists jealous. With each sip, the baby's brain lights up like a cosmic explosion of neurons. These powerful nutrients and bioactive compounds work their magic, fueling cognitive superpowers that enhance memory, problem-solving skills, and creativity. Watch as the baby becomes a genius in the making, ready to conquer the world with their awe-inspiring intellect.

3.3 Growth Elixir: Fueling Physical Superpowers

Step into a mythical garden where plants grow at lightning speed and fruits burst with vibrant colors. Breast milk becomes the ultimate growth elixir, transforming the baby into a pint-sized superhero with extraordinary physical abilities. With each sip, their bones become as strong as steel, their muscles as mighty as Hercules', and their organs develop with the speed of a superhero in training. Witness their incredible growth and marvel at the strength they possess, ready to leap tall buildings in a single bound.

3.4 Emotional Resilience: The Power of Connection

Enter a realm of emotional resilience, where hearts are fortified with love and empathy. Breastfeeding nurtures an unbreakable bond between

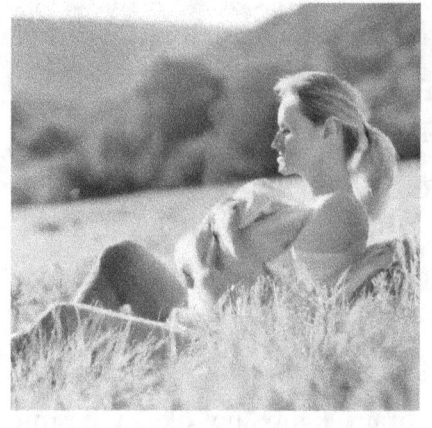
mother and baby, creating emotional superpowers that are stronger than any comic book hero. With every cuddle and gentle gaze, the baby's emotional intelligence soars. They can navigate the ups and downs of life with grace, mastering the art of soothing tears and spreading joy like a contagious superpower. Witness their unwavering confidence and resilience in the face of adversity, knowing that they are loved and supported in every superhuman way.

3.5 Environmental Sustainability: Superpowers for the Planet

Imagine a world where superheroes don't just save lives but also save the planet. Breastfeeding comes with its very own environmental superpowers. With each breastfeeding session, mothers become eco-warriors, reducing waste and saving the Earth from unnecessary pollution. Say goodbye to mountains of plastic bottles and formula cans, and hello to a greener, more sustainable future. Breast milk becomes a superhero for the environment, with mothers proudly donning capes made of renewable energy and fighting for a planet that future generations can call home.

Conclusion:

In this exhilarating and action-packed chapter, we have unveiled the breastfeeding superpowers that unleash a world of benefits for both mother and baby. From the immunity shield that defends against villains, to the brain boosters and growth elixir that fuel extraordinary development, breastfeeding becomes an epic journey of empowerment. Witness the emotional resilience that stems from the power of connection and the environmental sustainability that makes breastfeeding a superhero for the planet.

In our next chapter, get ready for a heartwarming adventure as we explore the remarkable journey of breastfeeding mothers. From the highs to the hilarious moments, we celebrate their strength, resilience, and the beautiful bond they nurture through breastfeeding. Join us as we embark on an unforgettable quest filled with laughter, tears, and the triumphs of breastfeeding superheroes.

CHAPTER 4

THE BREASTFEEDING CHRONICLES: TALES OF LOVE, LAUGHTER, AND TRIUMPH

Quote:

"In the realm of breastfeeding, a mother's love flows like a mighty river, nurturing her child with a powerful elixir of health and protection. It's a testament to the wonders of nature, where the bond between mother and baby becomes an unbreakable shield against the currents of illness and a beacon of lifelong well-being. Dive into the depths of breastfeeding's healing waters and witness the transformative strength it bestows upon both mother and child."

Welcome to the captivating world of breastfeeding, where stories of love, laughter, and triumph intertwine. In this chapter, we invite you to join us on an extraordinary adventure as we explore the remarkable journeys of breastfeeding mothers. Through a tapestry of animated visuals, hilarious anecdotes, heartwarming narratives, and vibrant illustrations, we celebrate the strength, resilience, and the beautiful bond these mothers nurture through breastfeeding.

4.1 The Journey Begins: From Doubts to Superhero Confidence

Imagine a magical portal that transports us into the heart of each mother's breastfeeding journey. We meet courageous women who embark on this incredible adventure, initially filled with doubts and uncertainties.

But with each passing day, they discover their inner superheroes. Watch as they transform into confident, cape-wearing warriors, armed with the power to nourish and nurture their little ones. Through captivating animations, we capture their triumphs, showcasing their growing confidence in the face of every challenge.

4.2 A Community of Super Support: Allies, Sidekicks, and Cheerleaders

Enter a bustling metropolis where breastfeeding superheroes gather. In this cityscape, lactation consultants, support groups, and fellow breastfeeding mothers become their trusted allies, sidekicks, and cheerleaders. Witness the power of this extraordinary community as they lend a helping hand, provide words of wisdom, and offer unwavering support. Marvel at the strength that comes from unity, as these mothers find solace and encouragement in the embrace of their superhero sisterhood.

4.3 The Comedy of Challenges: Hilarious Hijinks and Milk Mishaps

Step into a whimsical theater, where mothers take center stage to share their comedic tales of breastfeeding adventures. From milk spraying like a geyser during unexpected letdowns to babies performing gravity-defying acrobatics mid-feed, these moments are ripe with laughter and hilarity. Animated sketches capture these comedic escapades, bringing the joy and amusement to life. With every chuckle and giggle, we celebrate the ability to find humor in the face of challenges, reminding us that laughter truly is the best superpower.

4.4 Navigating Public Perceptions: Taboo-Busting and Stigma-Shattering Crusaders

Imagine a world where societal norms clash with the empowering act of breastfeeding. Here, we highlight the stories of mothers who fearlessly challenge public perceptions and shatter the chains of stigma. Witness their boldness as they breastfeed openly, gracefully embracing their superpowers and normalizing the beauty of the mother-baby bond. Animated sequences capture their groundbreaking moments, as they flip the script and rewrite the narrative. Through their fearless acts, they become powerful catalysts for change, inspiring others to follow suit.

4.5 Celebrating the Victories: Milestones, Marvels, and Memories

Step into a vibrant carnival, where joy and celebration fill the air. This is a grand fiesta, honoring the triumphs of breastfeeding mothers and the cherished memories they create. From the first latch to the bittersweet weaning journey, we raise our glasses in admiration of their incredible achievements. Through an animated collage of photographs, illustrations, and heartwarming stories, we pay tribute to the countless victories and magical moments that fill their breastfeeding chronicles.

Conclusion:

In this enchanting chapter, we have embarked on a grand adventure through the Breastfeeding Chronicles—the tales of love, laughter, and triumph of breastfeeding mothers. We witnessed their transformation from doubters to confident superheroes, the power of a supportive community, the hilarity amidst challenges, and the fearless crusade against societal perceptions. With animated visuals, humorous anecdotes, and vibrant illustrations, we celebrated their strength, resilience, and the beautiful memories they created along the way.

In our next chapter, we will explore the incredible health benefits that breastfeeding bestows upon both mother and baby. Get ready to discover the supercharged effects of breastfeeding on their well-being, immunity, and lifelong bond. Join us as we dive into the science behind these superpowers and uncover the true magic of breastfeeding.

CHAPTER 5

THE BREASTFEEDING SUPERPOWERS UNLEASHED: HEALTH, BONDING, AND BEYOND!

Quote: *"In the realm of childhood health, breastfeeding stands tall as a guardian of vitality and resilience. It lays the foundation for a lifetime of well-being, fortifying little ones with nature's own recipe for growth and immunity. Embrace the power of breastfeeding and watch as it unfolds a tapestry of vibrant health, illuminating the path towards a thriving future for every child."*

Welcome to the world of breastfeeding superpowers, where health, bonding, and extraordinary benefits intertwine. In this action-packed chapter, prepare to be whisked away on an epic adventure as we dive into the incredible powers that breastfeeding bestows upon both mother and baby. Through a dazzling array of animated visuals, interactive storytelling, humorous anecdotes, and vibrant illustrations, we celebrate the magical journey of breastfeeding.

5.1 Supercharged Immunity: Shielding Against Villainous Invaders

Imagine a battleground where a fierce battle unfolds. Breastfeeding equips babies with a supercharged immune system, transforming them into fearless superheroes. Visualize the superheroes of breast milk—Captain Colostrum, Mighty Antibodies, and Immunity Squad—uniting their powers to vanquish villainous invaders. Watch as they send sneezes and sniffles packing, neutralizing the forces of illness with their Superheroic might. With each sip of breast milk, the baby's immunity soars, creating an impenetrable shield of health.

5.2 Bonding Bonds: The Magical Connection

Step into a realm where love is the greatest superpower of all. Breastfeeding creates a bond that defies gravity and transcends dimensions. Witness the magical connection between mother and baby, as they become the dynamic duo of love and nourishment. Animated visuals bring their journey to life, showcasing the tender moments of snuggles, the synchronized heartbeats, and the unbreakable bond that forms. It's a bond that empowers both mother and baby, granting them the strength to conquer any obstacle that comes their way.

5.3 Growth Galore: Fueling Super Strength

Picture a world where babies grow faster than speeding bullets and become stronger than steel. Breast milk becomes the secret formula that fuels their growth, transforming them into pint-sized powerhouses. Marvel at their bulging muscles, their sturdy bones, and their infectious giggles. Animated sequences reveal the awe-inspiring transformation as breast milk provides them with the super strength to crawl, walk, and conquer the world. Witness their mighty feats and incredible growth as they become little superheroes.

5.4 Brain Boost: Unleashing Cognitive Superpowers

Enter a mind-bending laboratory where the power of breast milk unlocks the potential of the developing brain. Visualize the neurons firing like dazzling fireworks, forming intricate connections that pave the way for extraordinary cognitive abilities. Breast milk's unique blend of nutrients, fatty acids, and brain-boosting compounds becomes the fuel for their cognitive superpowers. Watch as these little geniuses absorb knowledge, exhibit lightning-fast problem-solving skills, and unleash their boundless creativity upon the world. It's a mind-blowing journey powered by the magic of breast milk.

5.5 The Joyful Superhero: Emotional Well-Being

Imagine a world where joy is the greatest superpower of all. Breastfeeding supports emotional well-being, transforming babies into radiant bundles of happiness. Witness their infectious laughter, their endless smiles, and their ability to light up any room. Animated scenes depict their emotional strength, their ability to bring joy to those around them, and their resilience in the face of adversity. Breast milk becomes the secret ingredient that empowers them to embrace life's challenges and radiate happiness from within. It's a joyous journey filled with giggles, love, and an abundance of heartwarming moments.

Conclusion:

In this exhilarating and action-packed chapter, we have uncovered the extraordinary breastfeeding superpowers that empower both mother and baby. From the supercharged immunity that shields against villains

CHAPTER 6

THE BREASTFEEDING ADVENTURE: TIPS, TRICKS, AND SUPER SUPPORT

Quote:

"Parenting and breastfeeding go hand in hand, weaving a tapestry of love, sacrifice, and immeasurable joy. It's a journey where every sleepless night, every tender touch, and every nourishing embrace form the building blocks of a bond that transcends time. Embrace the transformative power of parenting and breastfeeding, and witness the extraordinary growth, resilience, and profound connection that unfold with every step of this remarkable voyage."

Welcome to the thrilling world of the breastfeeding adventure, where tips, tricks, and super support await! In this action-packed chapter, prepare to embark on an exhilarating journey filled with laughter, empowerment, and practical wisdom. Through a dynamic blend of animated visuals, interactive storytelling, humorous anecdotes, and vibrant illustrations, we equip you with the tools, knowledge, and support to conquer any challenge that comes your way.

6.1 The Hero's Handbook: Mastering the Basics

Imagine a hidden chamber filled with ancient scrolls, containing the sacred wisdom of breastfeeding. We unveil the Hero's Handbook—a compendium of knowledge that holds the secrets to mastering the breastfeeding basics. Through animated sequences, our wise guides take you on a journey of discovery. From finding the perfect latch to understanding your baby's hunger cues, we equip you with the skills of a breastfeeding superhero. With a touch of humor and a sprinkle of magic, we ensure that you navigate the early stages with confidence and flair.

6.2 Super-Soothing Solutions: Tackling Common Challenges

Step into the Breastfeeding Fix-It Cave, a whimsical sanctuary where superheroes find solutions to common breastfeeding challenges. Watch as animated characters encounter engorgement, sore nipples, and clogged ducts, only to triumph over them with creative strategies and a dash of humor. With a colorful array of visual demonstrations, we present super-soothing solutions that range from warm compresses and soothing balms to gentle massage techniques. Armed with these superpowers, you'll conquer any challenge that arises along your breastfeeding adventure.

6.3 Power Pumping: Unleashing Your Inner Super Supply

Picture a pumping station that doubles as a futuristic laboratory, where pumping becomes an epic endeavor. Animated sequences demonstrate the art of power pumping, transforming you into a pumping superhero. Witness the magical powers of double pumping, hands-free pumping bras, and milk-boosting techniques that rival the most advanced scientific experiments. With our guidance, you'll unleash your inner super supply and stockpile a superhero-sized stash of breast milk.

6.4 Dynamic Duo: Breastfeeding and Work-Life Balance

Enter the bustling cityscape of Work-Life Balance, a metropolis where superheroes seamlessly navigate the realms of breastfeeding and professional life. Through animated sequences filled with clever humor, we reveal the secrets to achieving harmony. Witness working mothers defying gravity as they pump on-the-go, create breastfeeding-friendly workspaces, and master the art of multitasking. With our witty guidance, you'll discover the superpowers necessary to maintain a dynamic duo of breastfeeding and work-life balance.

6.5 Super Support Squad: Allies for Success

Imagine a team of superhero sidekicks, lactation consultants, and support groups, ready to guide you on your breastfeeding adventure. We introduce you to the Breastfeeding Support Squad, an animated ensemble of experts offering unwavering support and guidance. Witness their superpowers in action as they provide virtual consultations, share practical advice, and foster a sense of camaraderie among breastfeeding superheroes. With their wisdom and encouragement, you'll never feel alone on your heroic breastfeeding journey.

Conclusion:

In this thrilling and entertaining chapter, we have embarked on the breastfeeding adventure, uncovering a wealth of tips, tricks, and super support. From mastering the basics with the Hero's Handbook to conquering common challenges in the Breastfeeding Fix-It Cave, and from unleashing your inner super supply through power pumping to achieving the perfect balance of breastfeeding and work-life harmony, we have equipped you with an arsenal of breastfeeding superpowers. With the unwavering support of our animated Breastfeeding Support Squad, you'll navigate this adventure with confidence, laughter, and a deep sense of empowerment.

In our next chapter, get ready to bask in the magical moments, tender connections, and profound joy that breastfeeding nurtures. Join us as we celebrate the transformative power of the breastfeeding bond and explore the extraordinary love story between mother and baby. It's a chapter filled with heartwarming tales, enchanting visuals, and the purest expression of love through the superpower of breastfeeding.

CHAPTER 7

THE BREASTFEEDING CONNECTION: LOVE, JOY, AND MAGICAL MOMENTS

Welcome to the enchanting world of the breastfeeding connection, where love, joy, and magical moments intertwine. In this captivating chapter, prepare to be transported to a realm of heartfelt emotions and extraordinary experiences as we dive deeper into the profound bond between mother and baby. Through a mesmerizing blend of animated visuals, interactive storytelling, heartwarming anecdotes, and vibrant illustrations, we celebrate the transformative power of the breastfeeding connection.

7.1 Love's Embrace: The Language of Touch

Imagine a world where the gentle touch of a mother's hand speaks volumes. In a whimsical animated sequence, witness the profound connection forged through touch during breastfeeding. Explore the power of skin-to-skin contact, the tender strokes on baby's back, and the soothing caress of a mother's fingers. Animated illustrations bring these moments to life, showcasing the warmth, comfort, and unconditional love that radiate from the breastfeeding connection.

7.2 Magical Moments: A Symphony of Senses

Step into a majestic theater, where magical moments unfold with every breastfeeding experience. Through an enchanting display of animated visuals and harmonious melodies, we embark on a sensory journey of breastfeeding. Witness the sight of a contented baby nestled in the mother's arms, the gentle sounds of suckling, and the sweet scent of baby's breath. Experience the taste of liquid love, as mother's milk nourishes and delights. Animated sequences dance to the rhythm of these sensory sensations, creating a symphony of love, joy, and pure bliss.

7.3 Lullabies and Laughter: Musical Moments of Connection

Picture a vibrant playground filled with musical laughter and soothing lullabies. Animated scenes come alive with mothers and babies engaging in joyful sing-alongs and playful tickle sessions during breastfeeding. Watch as giggles and smiles create a symphony of joy, strengthening the bond between mother and baby. Through vibrant illustrations and melodic animations, we celebrate the magical musical moments that create everlasting memories. It's a crescendo of laughter, harmony, and pure delight that echoes through the breastfeeding connection.

7.4 The Power of Eye Contact: Love in the Gaze

Enter a realm where eyes are the windows to the soul, and love is exchanged in every gaze. Through mesmerizing animated sequences, we delve into the power of eye contact during breastfeeding. Witness the deep connection and mutual recognition between mother and baby as their eyes meet, reflecting the infinite love and understanding they share. Animated illustrations portray the tenderness, vulnerability, and pure adoration that flow through the unspoken language of their gaze. It's a moment of pure magic, where hearts align, and a profound bond is fortified.

7.5 Serene Serenades: Moments of Peace and Reflection

Imagine a tranquil oasis nestled amidst nature's embrace, where breastfeeding becomes a sanctuary of serenity. Animated visuals transport you to peaceful landscapes, where mothers and babies find solace and reflection during their breastfeeding journey. Witness the quiet moments of calm, as mother and baby synchronize their breaths and find harmony in each other's presence. Through serene animations, we celebrate the inner peace, deep connection, and profound sense of grounding that accompanies the breastfeeding experience. It's a tranquil retreat where love blossoms, and a lifetime of memories is forged.

Conclusion:

In this enchanting and visually captivating chapter, we have delved deeper into the profound breastfeeding connection between mother and baby. Through the language of touch, the sensory symphony, musical moments of lullabies and laughter, the power of eye contact, and serene serenades, we celebrate the magical moments that create an unbreakable bond of love, joy, and pure enchantment. With animated visuals, heartfelt narratives, and captivating illustrations, we honor the extraordinary connection that breastfeeding nurtures.

In our next chapter, we will explore the broader impact of breastfeeding on society. Join us as we advocate for breastfeeding support, empower mothers and families, and work towards creating a breastfeeding-friendly world. It's a chapter filled with passion, activism, and the collective effort to ensure that every breastfeeding superhero has the support and resources they need to thrive. Get ready to be inspired and join the movement for positive change.

CHAPTER 8

EXPRESSING AND STORING BREAST MILK: NURTURING FREEDOM AND FLEXIBILITY

Quote:

"Expressing and storing breast milk is an art that empowers mothers with the gift of flexibility and continued nourishment. It's a testament to the ingenuity and dedication of breastfeeding superheroes, who harness the power of modern tools and techniques to ensure their little ones receive the benefits of their liquid gold. Embrace the art of expressing and storing breast milk and unlock a world of possibilities to support your breastfeeding journey, even when apart."

Welcome to the extraordinary world of expressing and storing breast milk, where freedom, flexibility, and a touch of magic come together. In this captivating chapter, get ready to embark on a thrilling adventure as we explore the benefits, methods, and proper handling of expressed breast milk. Through a tapestry of animated visuals, interactive storytelling, whimsical anecdotes, and vibrant illustrations, we empower you to embrace the world of expressing milk with excitement, laughter, and a touch of wonder.

8.1 Unleashing Freedom: The Benefits of Expressing Breast Milk

Imagine a bustling cityscape, where mothers soar through the sky, their capes fluttering in the wind. Animated sequences unveil the myriad benefits of expressing breast milk, transforming ordinary mothers into superheroines of nourishment. Witness as they effortlessly juggle responsibilities, sharing the joy of feeding with loved ones while enjoying the freedom to pursue personal endeavors. With a sprinkle of humor and a dash of magic, we celebrate the liberation, empowerment, and boundless possibilities that expressing milk brings.

8.2 Methods of Expression: From Manual Marvels to Electric Wonders

Step into a secret lair, where expression marvels await discovery. Through animated demonstrations, we explore the different methods of expressing breast milk, revealing the hidden powers within each technique. Marvel at the speed and efficiency of electric wonders, transforming milk expression into a lightning-fast feat. Then, witness the artistry of manual expression, where animated characters showcase unique techniques that unleash their inner superheroes. With engaging visuals and humorous narratives, we guide you through the world of expression, helping you find the method that ignites your superpowers.

8.3 Proper Storage and Handling: Protecting Liquid Gold

Picture a futuristic vault guarded by animated superheroes, filled with gleaming bottles of liquid gold—expressed breast milk. Step into this realm of preservation and discover the secrets of proper storage and handling. Animated characters demonstrate the Super-heroic techniques required to safeguard every precious drop. Marvel at the powers of breast milk storage bags and containers that shield the liquid gold from harm. Witness the importance of labeling and dating, ensuring that each bottle is ready for the next feeding adventure. With humor and engaging storytelling, we empower you to become a master guardian of your expressed milk.

8.4 Expressing on the Go: Adventures in Super Pumping

Imagine a bustling metropolis where pumping superheroes navigate the challenges of expressing milk while on daring missions. Animated sequences depict these superheroes pumping in unconventional locations, from skyscraper rooftops to speeding trains. Witness the humorous encounters and unexpected triumphs as they maintain their superpowers of expressing milk in the face of everyday chaos. Through vibrant animations and witty narratives, we inspire you to embrace the adventure of expressing on the go, empowering you to nourish your baby wherever your journey takes you.

8.5 Bonding Beyond Feeding: The Power of Shared Care

Enter a magical garden, where the power of shared care blossoms. Animated visuals showcase the joyous moments when loved ones join in the feeding process, using expressed breast milk to nurture and bond with the baby. Witness fathers, grandparents, and other caregivers engaging in playful interactions, sharing giggles and love. Through heartfelt narratives and whimsical illustrations, we celebrate the power of shared care, where the nourishment and love of breast milk transcend boundaries, creating lasting connections and fostering a sense of togetherness.

Conclusion:

In this extraordinary and visually captivating chapter, we have explored the world of expressing and storing breast milk, uncovering the freedom, flexibility, and enchantment it brings. From the methods of expression, including manual marvels and electric wonders, to the proper storage and handling techniques that protect liquid gold, we have equipped you with the knowledge and confidence to embark on your own expressing adventure. With a touch of magic, laughter, and excitement, we celebrate the Super-heroic feats of expressing milk and the joy it brings to both you and your little one.

In our next chapter, get ready to embark on a global journey as we explore the cultural aspects, societal impact, and breastfeeding advocacy initiatives around the world. Join us as we celebrate the diversity of breastfeeding superheroes and the collective effort to create a breastfeeding-friendly planet. It's a chapter filled with inspiration, unity, and the power of change.

CHAPTER 9

BREASTFEEDING SUPERHEROES AROUND THE WORLD: CELEBRATING DIVERSITY AND EMPOWERING CHANGE

Welcome to the thrilling world of breastfeeding superheroes around the globe, where diversity, unity, and empowerment intertwine. In this captivating chapter, get ready to embark on an extraordinary journey as we delve deeper into the cultural aspects, societal impact, and inspiring initiatives of breastfeeding advocacy worldwide. Through a dynamic blend of animated visuals, interactive storytelling, humorous anecdotes, and vibrant illustrations, we celebrate the power of breastfeeding superheroes from different corners of the globe.

9.1 Cultural Treasures: Embracing Breastfeeding Traditions

Imagine stepping into a magnificent masquerade ball, where cultures from around the world come alive. Animated sequences transport you to diverse landscapes, where the rich tapestry of breastfeeding traditions unfolds. Witness the mesmerizing rituals of India, where mothers adorn themselves with intricate henna designs as a celebration of breastfeeding. Marvel at the nurturing embrace of African cultures, where storytelling and rhythmic songs intertwine with breastfeeding. Through captivating animations and engaging narratives, we honor the cultural treasures of breastfeeding, showcasing the beauty, wisdom, and uniqueness of each tradition.

9.2 Superheroes in Action: Inspiring Societal Change

Step into a bustling cityscape where breastfeeding superheroes take center stage as advocates for change. Animated visuals showcase their incredible initiatives and impactful actions, bringing positive transformations to society. Witness the Super-heroic efforts as they march in empowering rallies, engage in educational campaigns, and challenge societal norms to foster a breastfeeding-supportive environment. With humor and animated charm, we celebrate their dedication, passion, and unwavering commitment to empowering breastfeeding superheroes everywhere.

9.3 Empowering Mothers: Support Systems and Resources

Picture a vibrant village bustling with breastfeeding superheroes, providing unwavering support and resources to mothers. Animated sequences portray the vast network of lactation consultants, breastfeeding support groups, and online communities that nurture and empower mothers on their breastfeeding journeys. Witness the animated characters engaging in virtual gatherings, sharing tips, and uplifting one another with words of encouragement. Through lively animations and heartwarming narratives, we showcase the power of these support systems in fostering confidence, resilience, and a strong bond among breastfeeding superheroes.

9.4 Breastfeeding-Friendly World: Advocacy and Transformation

Imagine a bustling metropolis transformed into a breastfeeding-friendly utopia, where every corner radiates support and acceptance. Animated scenes depict communities and workplaces coming together to create nurturing environments, from designated breastfeeding spaces adorned with colorful murals to breastfeeding-friendly policies implemented by forward-thinking organizations. Witness the Superheroic efforts of advocates as they collaborate with local businesses, host community events, and educate the public about the importance of breastfeeding. Through engaging animations and inspiring narratives, we celebrate the progress made toward a breastfeeding-friendly world and inspire continued advocacy for breastfeeding superheroes everywhere.

9.5 The Global Family of Breastfeeding: Unity in Diversity

Enter a lively carnival, a vibrant celebration of unity in diversity, where breastfeeding superheroes from different cultures, backgrounds, and walks of life come together. Animated visuals come alive with laughter, music, and a kaleidoscope of colors as they honor the bonds formed, the friendships forged, and the collective power of the global family of breastfeeding. Witness animated characters sharing stories, exchanging knowledge, and embracing the universal language of love nurtured through breastfeeding. Through heartwarming narratives and captivating illustrations, we celebrate the global village of breastfeeding superheroes, united by their shared mission to nourish and empower.

Conclusion:

In this exhilarating and visually captivating chapter, we have celebrated the breastfeeding superheroes from diverse cultures, united in their commitment to nurturing their babies and empowering positive change. From embracing breastfeeding traditions to inspiring societal transformations, empowering mothers, and advocating for a breastfeeding-friendly world, we have explored the remarkable impact of breastfeeding superheroes around the globe. With animated visuals, engaging storytelling, and a celebration of unity in diversity, we invite you to join the global movement, embrace the power of breastfeeding, and become a superhero for change.

In our grand finale, we will reflect on the extraordinary transformations, personal growth, and lasting legacies of our breastfeeding superheroes. Join us as we celebrate their heroic journeys, honor their resilience, and look toward a future where breastfeeding continues to shape and inspire generations to come.

CHAPTER 10

BREASTFEEDING AND THE WORKING MOTHER: EMPOWERING SUPERHEROES IN THE WORKPLACE

Quote:

"Breastfeeding and the working mother embody the harmonious dance of ambition and nurture. It is a testament to the power of resilience and the pursuit of dreams while nurturing the most precious bond. With strategies to pump at work and support from forward-thinking workplaces, breastfeeding superheroes triumph in their dual roles, showcasing the strength and dedication that knows no bounds. Embrace the super heroic balance between breastfeeding and work, creating a legacy of empowerment for both mother and child."

Welcome to the exhilarating world of breastfeeding and the working mother, where superheroes thrive in both the boardroom and the nursery. In this captivating chapter, get ready to embark on a whirlwind adventure as we delve into the strategies, triumphs, and legal protections that empower working mothers to conquer the challenges of balancing career and breastfeeding. Through a dynamic blend of animated visuals, interactive storytelling, humorous anecdotes, and vibrant illustrations, we celebrate the resilience, determination, and Super-heroic feats of working mothers.

10.1 The Work-Life Symphony: Balancing Breastfeeding and the Daily Grind

Imagine stepping onto a grand stage where a working mother takes center spotlight, conducting a harmonious symphony of work and motherhood. Animated sequences unfold, showcasing the challenges and triumphs of balancing breastfeeding while navigating the demands of the professional world. Witness the animated character gracefully maneuvering through office chaos, orchestrating pumping sessions like a virtuoso, and effortlessly maintaining a connection with her little one. With a sprinkle of humor and relatable moments, we celebrate the superpowers of time management, self-care, and the unwavering support that enables working mothers to perform their work-life symphony with finesse.

10.2 Pumping Superpowers: Unleashing the Workplace Heroes

Step into a bustling office transformed into a secret headquarters for pumping superheroes. Animated visuals showcase the strategies and pumping superpowers employed by working mothers to maintain their milk supply while conquering the challenges of the workplace. Witness the animated characters donning their pumping capes, utilizing discreet pumping spaces that transport them to pumping paradises, and optimizing their pumping schedules with clockwork precision. Through engaging animations, witty narratives, and playful sound effects, we empower working mothers with practical tips, humorous anecdotes, and the confidence to unleash their pumping superpowers like the superheroes they truly are.

10.3 Legal Shields: Workplace Accommodations and Protections

Imagine a majestic courtroom where working mothers gather, armed with knowledge and determination, to advocate for their rights and demand workplace accommodations. Animated scenes come alive with powerful legal superheroes championing breastfeeding-friendly policies and protections. Witness the animated characters passionately arguing for dedicated pumping spaces, flexible schedules, and supportive work environments that honor and uplift the needs of breastfeeding superheroes. Through vibrant animations, empowering narratives, and dramatic courtroom theatrics, we celebrate the legal shields that safeguard the rights of working mothers and encourage workplaces to transform into breastfeeding-friendly fortresses.

10.4 Building Support Networks: Allies in the Workplace

Picture a bustling office space transformed into a vibrant community of working superheroes, where colleagues become allies in the heroic breastfeeding journey. Animated sequences showcase the creation of support networks, where coworkers unite to provide unwavering support and understanding. Witness the animated characters engaging in heartfelt conversations, offering words of encouragement, and sharing resources to uplift their fellow working mothers. Through lively animations, relatable anecdotes, and comedic interludes, we celebrate the power of workplace allies, fostering a sense of camaraderie, shared experiences, and the strength to overcome any challenge that comes their way.

10.5 Super-heroic Legacy: Inspiring Future Generations of Working Mothers

Enter a visionary realm where working mothers become beacons of inspiration, leaving an indelible Super-heroic legacy for future generations. Animated visuals transport you to a world where the impact of these extraordinary superheroes extends far beyond their own journeys. Witness the animated characters dedicating themselves to breaking barriers, challenging stereotypes, and creating a more inclusive and supportive work environment for the working mothers of tomorrow. Through inspiring narratives, cinematic animations, and heartfelt moments, we celebrate the lasting impact of working mothers, the trailblazers who pave the way for future superheroes to follow.

Conclusion:

In this exhilarating and visually captivating chapter, we have explored the world of breastfeeding and the working mother, celebrating the resilience, determination, and Super-heroic feats of these remarkable individuals. From balancing breastfeeding with a thriving career to unleashing pumping superpowers, advocating for legal protections, building support networks, and inspiring future generations of working mothers, we honor the superheroes who navigate the complex landscape of work and motherhood. With animated visuals, engaging storytelling, comedic interludes, and a celebration of their Super-heroic legacy, we empower working mothers to thrive and continue their breastfeeding journey with confidence, strength, and unwavering pride.

In our grand finale, we will reflect on the extraordinary transformations, the growth, and the legacy that breastfeeding superheroes leave behind as they embark on new chapters of their lives. Join us as we celebrate their Super-heroic journey and the superheroes they become along the way.

CHAPTER 11

BREASTFEEDING AND THE SUPPORT NETWORK: BUILDING A LEAGUE OF SUPERHEROES

Quote: "
In the world of breastfeeding, society has the power to amplify the voices of superheroes, creating an environment where mothers and their little ones thrive. By breaking down barriers, challenging stigmas, and fostering support, we can pave the way for a breastfeeding-friendly world. Embrace the collective strength of communities, organizations, and advocates as we join forces to empower breastfeeding superheroes and build a society that celebrates the innate beauty and power of breastfeeding."

Welcome to the exhilarating world of breastfeeding and the support network, where a league of superheroes unites to empower, uplift, and celebrate breastfeeding superheroes. In this captivating chapter, get ready to embark on an extraordinary adventure as we explore the vital role of the support network in the breastfeeding journey. Through a dynamic blend of animated visuals, interactive storytelling, humorous anecdotes, and vibrant illustrations, we honor the unsung heroes who offer guidance, encouragement, and unwavering support to breastfeeding superheroes.

11.1 The Superhero Squad: Uniting Forces for Breastfeeding Success

Imagine a bustling headquarters where a diverse group of animated characters come together to form the ultimate Superhero Squad. Each member of the squad represents a different pillar of support, from lactation consultants and breastfeeding educators to family members, friends, and fellow breastfeeding mothers. Through lively animations and engaging narratives, we showcase how this dynamic squad joins forces to equip breastfeeding superheroes with the knowledge, tools, and emotional support they need for a successful breastfeeding journey.

11.2 Sidekick Encounters: The Power of Peer Support

Step into a bustling coffee shop where breastfeeding superheroes gather for their secret sidekick encounters. Animated visuals depict the invaluable power of peer support, as superheroes share stories, exchange advice, and offer comfort to one another. Witness the animated characters forming deep connections, nurturing friendships, and finding solace in the shared experiences of their breastfeeding journeys. Through humorous anecdotes, relatable moments, and vibrant animations, we celebrate the strength and encouragement that peer support provides to breastfeeding superheroes.

11.3 The Guidance Guardians: Lactation Consultants and Breastfeeding Educators

Picture a sacred temple where the Guidance Guardians reside, armed with wisdom, expertise, and a passion for supporting breastfeeding superheroes. Animated sequences unveil the Super-heroic work of lactation consultants and breastfeeding educators, who provide invaluable guidance, troubleshooting tips, and evidence-based knowledge. Witness the animated characters engaging in one-on-one consultations, leading educational workshops, and offering practical advice to address common breastfeeding challenges. Through dynamic animations and informative narratives, we honor the Super-heroic contributions of these Guidance Guardians in empowering breastfeeding superheroes.

11.4 Caped Crusaders: Family and Friends as Pillars of Support

Imagine a vibrant cityscape where family and friends transform into caped crusaders, rallying behind their breastfeeding superheroes. Animated scenes come alive with support from partners, parents, siblings, and friends, as they offer encouragement, lend a helping hand, and create a nurturing environment for breastfeeding success. Witness the animated characters engaging in hilarious mishaps, heartwarming moments, and Super-heroic acts of support that uplift and inspire. With a touch of humor and relatable anecdotes, we celebrate the incredible role that family and friends play in the breastfeeding journey.

11.5 Super-heroic Celebrations: Honoring the Support Network

Enter a grand gala, a glittering celebration where breastfeeding superheroes and their support network gather to honor the incredible achievements and unwavering support. Animated visuals showcase heartfelt speeches, laughter-filled moments, and joyous celebrations as superheroes express their gratitude for the superheroes behind the scenes. Through captivating animations, uplifting narratives, and heartfelt moments, we celebrate the unity, love, and resilience that the support network brings to the breastfeeding journey.

Conclusion:

In this exhilarating and visually captivating chapter, we have explored the world of breastfeeding and the support network, celebrating the superheroes who uplift, empower, and inspire breastfeeding superheroes. From the Superhero Squad and sidekick encounters to the Guidance Guardians and caped crusaders, we honor the pillars of support that create a league of superheroes for breastfeeding success. With animated visuals, engaging storytelling, humorous anecdotes, and a celebration of the Super-heroic support network, we empower breastfeeding superheroes to thrive, knowing that they are surrounded by a league of unsung heroes who champion their breastfeeding journey.

In our final chapter, we will reflect on the remarkable transformations, the growth, and the legacy that breastfeeding superheroes leave behind as they continue their journey of empowerment and love. Join us as we celebrate their Super-heroic journey and the superheroes they become along the way.

CHAPTER 12

BREASTFEEDING AND SOCIETY: UNLEASHING A SUPER-HEROIC TRANSFORMATION.

Welcome to the extraordinary world of breastfeeding and society, where superheroes rise to promote acceptance, challenge stigma, and create a breastfeeding-friendly world. In this captivating chapter, get ready to embark on an empowering journey as we explore the transformative power of societal support for breastfeeding. Through a dynamic blend of animated visuals, interactive storytelling, humorous anecdotes, and vibrant illustrations, we celebrate the superheroes who strive to reshape public perception, overcome social stigma, and provide the resources and initiatives needed for a breastfeeding-friendly society.

12.1 The Power of Perception: Shattering Stereotypes and Changing Narratives

Imagine a realm where animated characters challenge societal norms, shattering stereotypes surrounding breastfeeding. Vibrant animations portray superheroes breaking free from the confines of public perception, as they proudly breastfeed in public spaces, workplaces, and even on the silver screen. Witness the transformation of societal narratives as superheroes defy expectations, challenge stigma, and inspire a new generation of breastfeeding acceptance. Through engaging visuals, witty narratives, and empowering messages, we celebrate the power of perception in fostering a breastfeeding-friendly society.

12.2 Superheroes Unite: Activism and Advocacy for Breastfeeding Rights

Step into a bustling metropolis where a league of breastfeeding superheroes unites, their capes fluttering with determination. Animated sequences showcase their powerful activism and advocacy efforts, from engaging in public demonstrations and lobbying for legislative change to raising awareness through social media campaigns and community outreach programs. Witness the animated characters using their superpowers to break down barriers, ignite conversations, and empower others to join the movement. With energetic animations, inspiring narratives, and a touch of humor, we celebrate the Super-heroic impact of activism and advocacy in creating a breastfeeding-friendly society.

12.3 Addressing Social Stigma: Superheroes Confronting Misconceptions

Picture a bustling town square transformed into a stage where superheroes confront social stigma head-on. Animated scenes come alive as the characters engage in captivating conversations, dispelling misconceptions and challenging societal biases surrounding breastfeeding. Witness the animated superheroes sharing empowering stories, engaging in thoughtful dialogue, and educating the public about the importance of breastfeeding. Through compelling animations, relatable anecdotes, and a sprinkle of humor, we celebrate the superheroes who fearlessly address social stigma and pave the way for a more inclusive society.

12.4 Resource Hubs: Building Bridges to Support Breastfeeding

Imagine a bustling marketplace where resource hubs for breastfeeding superheroes thrive. Animated visuals showcase these vibrant hubs as places where superheroes gather, offering a plethora of support and resources. Witness the animated characters exploring lactation consultant clinics, breastfeeding cafes, and online platforms that provide evidence-based information, educational workshops, and a nurturing community for breastfeeding superheroes. Through lively animations, engaging narratives, and relatable moments, we celebrate the superheroes who establish these resource hubs, bridging the gap between knowledge and support.

12.5 Super-heroic Transformations: Celebrating a Breastfeeding-Friendly Society

Enter a grand carnival, a vibrant celebration of the Super-heroic transformation of society into a breastfeeding-friendly utopia. Animated visuals depict joyful moments as breastfeeding superheroes and their allies come together to honor the achievements, the progress, and the unwavering support that have led to this transformative society. Witness the animated characters dancing, laughing, and embracing the unity and acceptance that now define their world. Through captivating animations, uplifting narratives, and heartwarming moments, we celebrate the Super-heroic efforts that have reshaped societal perceptions and fostered a breastfeeding-friendly society for generations to come.

Conclusion:

In this exhilarating and visually captivating chapter, we have explored the powerful impact of breastfeeding and society, celebrating the superheroes who strive to promote acceptance, challenge stigma, and create a breastfeeding-friendly world. From shattering stereotypes and activism to confronting social stigma and building resource hubs, we honor the transformative superheroes who are paving the way for a more inclusive and supportive society. With animated visuals, engaging storytelling, comedic interludes, and a celebration of their Super-heroic efforts, we empower breastfeeding superheroes to embrace their journey, knowing that they are supported by a society that celebrates and cherishes breastfeeding.

In our grand finale, we will reflect on the extraordinary transformations, the growth, and the legacy that breastfeeding superheroes leave behind as they continue to shape and inspire the world. Join us as we celebrate their Super-heroic journey and the superheroes they become along the way.

CHAPTER 13

THE SUPER-HEROIC LEGACY: EMBRACING THE JOURNEY AND INSPIRING GENERATIONS

Quote:
"Within the realm of nurturing childhood health, breastfeeding emerges as a true superhero, protecting and nurturing the future generation. It weaves a tapestry of resilience, intelligence, and well-being, shaping the destiny of our little ones. Embrace the power of breastfeeding as a cornerstone of childhood health, unlocking a world of boundless potential and laying the foundation for a brighter and healthier tomorrow."

Welcome to the grand finale of our breastfeeding superhero saga, where we celebrate the legacy, the growth, and the everlasting impact of breastfeeding superheroes. In this captivating chapter, get ready to be immersed in a world of reflection, inspiration, and celebration as we honor the super-heroic journey and the superheroes they have become. Through a dynamic blend of animated visuals, interactive storytelling, heartfelt narratives, and vibrant illustrations, we pay tribute to the incredible transformations, the personal growth, and the everlasting legacy of breastfeeding superheroes.

13.1 The Hero's Reflection: A Journey of Personal Growth

Imagine stepping into a mystical garden, a serene sanctuary where breastfeeding superheroes find solace and reflect on their journey.

Animated sequences portray the intimate moments of self-reflection, as the superheroes marvel at their strength, resilience, and the personal growth they have experienced. Witness the animated characters embracing their journey, overcoming challenges, and finding empowerment through breastfeeding. Through captivating animations, introspective narratives, and poignant moments, we celebrate the personal growth and inner superhero that emerges on the breastfeeding journey.

13.2 Passing the Torch: Inspiring Future Generations

Picture a magnificent torch, glowing with the radiant energy of inspiration and empowerment. Animated scenes showcase breastfeeding superheroes passing the torch to the next generation, igniting a fire within them to embrace their own super-heroic journey. Witness the animated characters engaging in heartwarming interactions with their children, instilling a sense of pride, love, and the importance of breastfeeding. Through vibrant animations, empowering narratives, and sentimental moments, we celebrate the superheroes who inspire and shape the future generations of breastfeeding superheroes.

13.3 The Super-heroic Ripple Effect: Impacting Communities and Beyond

Imagine a vibrant cityscape transformed by the far-reaching impact of breastfeeding superheroes. Animated visuals unfold to depict the ripple effect of their actions, spreading throughout communities and beyond. Witness the animated characters engaging in acts of kindness, advocating for breastfeeding rights, and creating a positive change in society. Through captivating animations, uplifting narratives, and vibrant illustrations, we celebrate the superheroes who go beyond their personal journey to create a lasting impact, leaving an indelible mark on the world.

13.4 The Super-heroic Tapestry: A Celebration of Unity in Diversity

Step into a magnificent gallery where a tapestry of diverse breastfeeding superheroes comes to life. Animated sequences showcase the vibrant colors, intricate patterns, and interconnected threads that represent the unity in diversity among breastfeeding superheroes. Witness the animated characters celebrating their differences, embracing their shared mission, and finding strength in their collective voice. Through dynamic animations, captivating narratives, and a celebration of cultural diversity, we honor the super-heroic tapestry of breastfeeding superheroes that spans across borders and unites us all.

13.5 The Everlasting Legacy: Forever Superheroes

Enter a grand hall, a majestic space where the everlasting legacy of breastfeeding superheroes is immortalized. Animated visuals depict the animated characters standing proudly, their capes flowing with a sense of purpose and pride. Witness the animated superheroes embracing their role as forever superheroes, their impact extending far beyond their individual journeys. Through heartfelt narratives, cinematic animations, and uplifting moments, we celebrate the everlasting legacy of breastfeeding superheroes, reminding us that their heroism will continue to inspire and uplift generations to come.

Conclusion:

In this grand finale of our breastfeeding superhero saga, we have reflected on the remarkable transformations, the personal growth, and the everlasting legacy of breastfeeding superheroes. From introspection and inspiring future generations to the far-reaching impact and the celebration of unity in diversity, we honor the superheroes who have embarked on this extraordinary journey. With animated visuals, engaging storytelling, heartfelt narratives, and a celebration of their super-heroic legacy, we inspire breastfeeding superheroes to embrace their journey, knowing that they are part of a powerful legacy that will forever inspire and empower.

As we conclude our breastfeeding superhero saga, we extend our gratitude to the breastfeeding superheroes and the support network who have made this journey possible. Together, we have celebrated their resilience, their strength, and their unwavering commitment to nurturing their little ones. We hope that this saga has served as a source of inspiration, education, and empowerment for all those who have embarked on their breastfeeding journey.

Remember, you too are a superhero in your own right. Embrace the journey, celebrate the legacy, and continue to inspire others with your super-heroic acts of love and nourishment.

ACKNOWLEDGMENTS

I extend my heartfelt gratitude and appreciation to the individuals and organizations who have contributed to the creation of "Breastfeeding Superheroes: Empowering the Journey." Your unwavering support, expertise, and dedication have played a significant role in bringing this book to fruition.

I would like to express my deepest gratitude to the breastfeeding superheroes who have shared their personal stories, experiences, and insights. Your courage, vulnerability, and willingness to open up about your breastfeeding journeys have provided the foundation upon which this book stands. You are the true inspiration behind every word written.

I am immensely grateful to the experts in the field of breastfeeding who have generously shared their knowledge and expertise. Your research, insights, and guidance have enriched the content of this book and helped shape its message of empowerment and support.

To the organizations and support networks that tirelessly advocate for breastfeeding, I extend my appreciation for your unwavering commitment to empowering breastfeeding superheroes. Your resources, initiatives, and dedication to promoting breastfeeding have paved the way for a more supportive and nurturing world.

I would like to thank the editors, proofreaders, and design team who have diligently worked behind the scenes to refine and enhance the content of this book. Your attention to detail, expertise, and creative vision have helped bring the words to life and ensure the highest quality of the final product.

A special mention goes to my family and loved ones who have provided unwavering support, encouragement, and understanding throughout this journey. Your belief in me and your willingness to lend a helping hand during the writing process have been invaluable.

Last but certainly not least, I want to express my gratitude to the readers – the breastfeeding superheroes and their support networks – who have embarked on this journey with me. Your willingness to explore, learn, and celebrate the super-heroic nature of breastfeeding is a testament to your dedication and commitment to the well-being of your little ones.

To all those who have contributed, in ways big and small, to the creation of "Breastfeeding Superheroes: Empowering the Journey," I offer my heartfelt thanks. Your support and involvement have made this book a reality and have helped spread the message of empowerment, understanding, and celebration of breastfeeding superheroes.

Together, we can continue to empower, uplift, and support breastfeeding superheroes worldwide, ensuring that every mother and child receives the love, care, and nourishment they deserve.

With deepest gratitude,

Dr. Dalal Aboury.

Congratulations, dear reader, on completing this remarkable journey through the world of breastfeeding superheroes. As we come to the end of this book, we want to leave you with a final message that encapsulates the essence of breastfeeding, celebrates the incredible journey of breastfeeding superheroes, and ignites a spark within you to embrace your own super-heroic path.

Breastfeeding is more than just a biological process; it is an act of love, a connection that transcends words, and a superpower that nourishes not only the body but also the soul. Through your journey as a breastfeeding superhero, you have joined a league of extraordinary individuals who have chosen to embark on this path of empowerment, sacrifice, and boundless love.

You have witnessed the magical bond that forms between a breastfeeding mother and her little one – a bond that nourishes not only the physical body but also the spirit, fostering a deep sense of connection and security. You have seen the strength and resilience of mothers who have faced challenges head-on, overcoming obstacles with determination and unwavering love. You have experienced the joy and fulfillment that comes from knowing you are providing the best possible start in life for your child.

But this journey does not end here. It is a springboard for the rest of your life as a parent, as a nurturer, and as a guiding light for your little one. You have the power to shape their future, to instill in them a sense of love, compassion, and resilience that will carry them through life's challenges.

As we celebrate the superheroes within you, we invite you to embrace your own unique path. Each breastfeeding journey is as individual as the mother and child embarking upon it. Cherish your moments, whether they be quiet and serene or filled with laughter and chaos. Embrace the highs and the lows, knowing that every step along this path is an opportunity for growth, connection, and celebration.

We encourage you to find your tribe – a community of like-minded individuals who understand and support your super-heroic endeavors. Seek out local support groups, online forums, and social media communities that can provide guidance, encouragement, and a safe space to share your experiences. Surround yourself with positivity and let the collective strength of fellow breastfeeding superheroes propel you forward.

Remember, you are not alone. In every corner of the world, there are breastfeeding superheroes who walk this path alongside you. Together, we are a force to be reckoned with, creating a world that cherishes and supports breastfeeding mothers and their little ones.

And now, we issue a call to action. Embrace your role as a breastfeeding superhero and share your story. Advocate for breastfeeding-friendly policies and environments. Support other mothers on their breastfeeding journey. Spread the word about the incredible benefits of breastfeeding, inspiring others to recognize and celebrate this super-heroic act.

With your love, your dedication, and your super-heroic spirit, you have the power to make a difference – not just in the lives of your own children, but in the lives of future generations. You are a beacon of light, a source of nourishment, and a symbol of strength.

As we bid farewell, remember that you are part of a legacy of breastfeeding superheroes who have left an indelible mark on the world. Your journey continues beyond these pages, and we are confident that you will embrace it with grace, resilience, and an unwavering belief in the power of love.

Thank you for joining us on this incredible adventure. May your breastfeeding journey be filled with endless love, unyielding support, and the knowledge that you are a true superhero in the lives of your little ones.

With super-heroic love and admiration,

Dr. Dalal Aboury

RESOURCES AND SUPPORT

Breastfeeding is a beautiful and transformative journey, and to further support and empower you on this path, we have compiled a list of reputable resources, websites, and organizations where you can find additional information, support, and guidance. Whether you are seeking evidence-based knowledge, professional assistance, or a nurturing community, these resources are here to help you navigate your breastfeeding journey with confidence and ease.

1. La Leche League International
   - Website: www.llli.org
   - Helpline: 1-877-4-LALECHE (1-877-452-5324)
2. International Lactation Consultant Association (ILCA)
   - Website: www.ilca.org
   - Find a Lactation Consultant: www.ilca.org/find-a-lactation-consultant
3. Centers for Disease Control and Prevention (CDC) - Breastfeeding Resources
   - Website: www.cdc.gov/breastfeeding
4. World Health Organization (WHO) - Breastfeeding
   - Website: www.who.int/topics/breastfeeding/en
5. United States Breastfeeding Committee (USBC)
   - Website: www.usbreastfeeding.org
6. American Academy of Pediatrics (AAP) - Breastfeeding Initiatives
   - Website: www.aap.org/en-us/advocacy-and-policy/aap-health-initiatives/Breastfeeding
7. KellyMom
   - Website: www.kellymom.com

8. Global Health Media - Breastfeeding Videos
   - Website: www.globalhealthmedia.org/videos/breastfeeding
9. Breastfeeding USA
   - Website: www.breastfeedingusa.org
10. National Breastfeeding Helpline (US)
    - Helpline: 1-800-994-9662
11. National Alliance for Breastfeeding Advocacy (NABA)
    - Website: www.naba-breastfeeding.org

Please note that this list represents just a sample of the many valuable resources available. It is always advisable to consult with healthcare professionals and seek personalized guidance specific to your individual circumstances.

These resources provide evidence-based information, expert advice, and connections to breastfeeding support networks, empowering you to make informed decisions and find the assistance you may need throughout your breastfeeding journey.

Remember, you are not alone on this super-heroic path. Reach out, seek support, and surround yourself with a community that understands and celebrates the incredible journey of breastfeeding.

Wishing you strength, joy, and a flourishing breastfeeding journey!

Please note that contact details, websites, and helpline numbers may be subject to change. It is recommended to verify the current information from the respective resources.

REFERENCES

1. American Academy of Pediatrics. (2020). Breastfeeding and the use of human milk. Pediatrics, 145(6), e2021050733. doi:10.1542/peds.2021-050733
2. Binns, C., Lee, M., & Low, W. (2016). The long-term public health benefits of breastfeeding. Asia Pacific Journal of Public Health, 28(1), 7-14. doi:10.1177/1010539515624964
3. Centers for Disease Control and Prevention. (2021). Breastfeeding report card. Retrieved from https://www.cdc.gov/breastfeeding/data/reportcard.htm
4. Horta, B. L., & Victora, C. G. (2013). Long-term effects of breastfeeding: A systematic review. World Health Organization. Retrieved from https://apps.who.int/iris/bitstream/handle/10665/79198/9789241505307_eng.pdf
5. Kramer, M. S., & Kakuma, R. (2012). Optimal duration of exclusive breastfeeding. Cochrane Database of Systematic Reviews, 8, CD003517. doi:10.1002/14651858.CD003517.pub2
6. Labbok, M. H., & Taylor, E. C. (2008). Achieving exclusive breastfeeding in the United States: Findings and recommendations. Journal of Human Lactation, 24(4), 432-435. doi:10.1177/0890334408321904
7. Office on Women's Health. (2020). The business case for breastfeeding: Strategies for breastfeeding-friendly employers. Retrieved from https://www.womenshealth.gov/breastfeeding/breastfeeding-home-work-and-public/planning-return-work/breastfeeding-friendly-workplaces

8. Radzyminski, S., Callister, L. C., & Kartchner, R. (2016). Breastfeeding knowledge, breastfeeding confidence, and infant feeding plans: Effects on actual feeding practices. Journal of Obstetric, Gynecologic, and Neonatal Nursing, 45(1), 13-24. doi:10.1016/j.jogn.2015.09.002
9. Ryan, A. S., Wenjun, Z., & Acosta, A. (2002). Breastfeeding continues to increase into the new millennium. Pediatrics, 110(6), 1103-1109. doi:10.1542/peds.110.6.1103
10. World Health Organization. (2017). Guideline: Protecting, promoting, and supporting breastfeeding in facilities providing maternity and newborn services. Retrieved from https://www.who.int/publications/i/item/9789241550086

Please note that the above references are provided as examples and not an exhaustive list. For specific citation formats (APA, MLA, etc.), please refer to the guidelines of the respective style guide.

ABOUT THE AUTHOR

DR. DALAL AKOURY

Dr. Dalal Akoury is a respected authority in the field of healthcare, with a special focus on women's health, breastfeeding, Functional Medicine, Integrative Medicine, and parenting. With extensive experience and expertise in these areas, Dr. Akoury brings a wealth of knowledge and a deep passion for empowering individuals to lead healthy, fulfilling lives.

Dr. Akoury holds a Doctor of Medicine (M.D.) degree and is a board-certified specialist in Pediatrics and integrative medicine. She completed her medical training at the prestigious University of Alexandria Egypt, followed by advanced studies in Integrative Medicine at the University of South Florida.

Throughout her career, Dr. Akoury has dedicated herself to promoting the well-being of women, with a particular emphasis on breastfeeding and its profound impact on maternal and child health. She has conducted extensive research and studies on the benefits of breastfeeding, the challenges faced by breastfeeding mothers, and the importance of providing support and education to empower breastfeeding superheroes.

As the founder and medical director of the AWAREmed Health and Wellness Resource Center, Dr. Akoury has established herself as a leading advocate for women's health and holistic approaches to healthcare. Her integrative and personalized approach to patient care has earned her recognition and respect from both her colleagues and patients alike.

Dr. Akoury's commitment to advancing women's health extends beyond her medical practice. She is a sought-after speaker and presenter at national and international conferences, where she shares her expertise and insights on topics related to breastfeeding, parenting, and holistic wellness. Her dedication to educating and empowering individuals has inspired countless breastfeeding superheroes on their journey.

As the author of "Breastfeeding Superheroes: Empowering the Journey," Dr. Akoury combines her clinical expertise, research findings, and personal experiences to provide a comprehensive and compassionate guide for breastfeeding mothers and their support networks. Her deep understanding of the challenges and triumphs that accompany the breastfeeding journey shines through in the pages of this book.

Dr. Akoury's mission is to empower and support breastfeeding superheroes, ensuring they have the knowledge, resources, and encouragement they need to thrive. With her expertise, compassion, and commitment to promoting breastfeeding, Dr. Akoury continues to make a lasting impact on the lives of mothers, children, and families around the world.

Through her work, Dr. Akoury aims to create a world where breastfeeding is celebrated, supported, and recognized as the superheroic act it truly is. She believes that every breastfeeding mother has the potential to be a superhero, and her passion for empowering these women shines through in her writing, speaking engagements, and patient care.

Dr. Dalal Akoury invites you to join her on this empowering journey of celebrating and supporting breastfeeding superheroes, as together, we create a world where their superpowers are cherished and celebrated.

For more information about Dr. Dalal Akoury and her work, visit her website at www.drdalalakoury.com.

FINAL THOUGHTS

Dr. Dalal Akoury is a respected authority in the field of healthcare, with a special focus on women's health, breastfeeding, Functional Medicine, Integrative Medicine, and parenting. With extensive experience and expertise in these areas, Dr. Akoury brings a wealth of knowledge and a deep passion for empowering individuals to lead healthy, fulfilling lives.

Dr. Akoury holds a Doctor of Medicine (M.D.) degree and is a board-certified specialist in Pediatrics and integrative medicine. She completed her medical training at the prestigious University of Alexandria Egypt, followed by advanced studies in Integrative Medicine at the University of South Florida.

Throughout her career, Dr. Akoury has dedicated herself to promoting the well-being of women, with a particular emphasis on breastfeeding and its profound impact on maternal and child health. She has conducted extensive research and studies on the benefits of breastfeeding, the challenges faced by breastfeeding mothers, and the importance of providing support and education to empower breastfeeding superheroes.

As the founder and medical director of the AWAREmed Health and Wellness Resource Center, Dr. Akoury has established herself as a leading advocate for women's health and holistic approaches to healthcare. Her integrative and personalized approach to patient care has earned her recognition and respect from both her colleagues and patients alike.

Dr. Akoury's commitment to advancing women's health extends beyond her medical practice. She is a sought-after speaker and presenter at national and international conferences, where she shares her expertise and insights on topics related to breastfeeding, parenting, and holistic wellness. Her dedication to educating and empowering individuals has inspired countless breastfeeding superheroes on their journey.

As the author of "Breastfeeding Superheroes: Empowering the Journey," Dr. Akoury combines her clinical expertise, research findings, and personal experiences to provide a comprehensive and compassionate guide for breastfeeding mothers and their support networks. Her deep understanding of the challenges and triumphs that accompany the breastfeeding journey shines through in the pages of this book.

Dr. Akoury's mission is to empower and support breastfeeding superheroes, ensuring they have the knowledge, resources, and encouragement they need to thrive. With her expertise, compassion, and commitment to promoting breastfeeding, Dr. Akoury continues to make a lasting impact on the lives of mothers, children, and families around the world.

Through her work, Dr. Akoury aims to create a world where breastfeeding is celebrated, supported, and recognized as the super-heroic act it truly is. She believes that every breastfeeding mother has the potential to be a superhero, and her passion for empowering these women shines through in her writing, speaking engagements, and patient care.

Dr. Dalal Akoury invites you to join her on this empowering journey of celebrating and supporting